CN00942136

The Complete Keto Diet Weight Loss Cookbook

Quick and Delicious Recipes for Every
Day incl. Desserts, Side Dishes and More

Matthew Bailey

Copyright © [2021] [Matthew Bailey]

All rights reserved

All rights for this book here presented belong exclusively to the author.
Usage or reproduction of the text is forbidden and requires a clear consent of the author in case of expectations.

ISBN- 9798732105759

Table of Contents

Introduction

The keto diet is one of the prevalent and recognized diet plans worldwide. Keto diet or Ketogenic is a term used to describe a low-carb diet. It is also synonymous with the Atkins diet or low-carb diet.

The ketogenic diet can be traced back to many centuries ago. The idea is to have a diet plan that comprises more protein and fat and fewer carbohydrates. Precisely, when undertaking a keto diet plan, the foods that you should take must contain high amounts of fat, a moderate amount of protein, and a limited amount of carbs.

An average keto diet comprises at least 70 per cent of calories derived from fat, less than 10 per cent from carbs, and less than 20 per cent from protein. Similarly, Pamela Nisevich Bede, a dietitian with Abbott's EAS Sports Nutrition in Columbus, Ohio, America, says that the food eaten daily in the keto diet should be broken down to 75 per cent of fat, 20 per cent of protein, and 5 per cent of carbohydrates of your daily calories. This type of diet helps you to burn fat more effectively.

The keto diet is a diet that causes the body to release ketones into the bloodstream. Foods included in the keto diet include meats, eggs, processed meats, sausages, cheeses, fish, nuts, butter, oils, seeds, and fibrous vegetables. Usually, due to its restrictive nature, it is difficult to see through in the long run. Our regular diet is generally filled up with more Carbohydrates.

The ketogenic diet aims to enter a state of ketosis through fat metabolism. When the body is in a ketogenic state, carbohydrate is substituted for fat when energy is to be used. It is the state where your body does not have enough carbs for the cells to use. With low levels of carbohydrates, fat can be converted to ketones in the liver, which are used to fuel the body. This usually happens after following the diet plan strictly for a couple of days. If you are attempting the keto diet for the first time, you might find this experience strange. Some signs make you aware that you are already in ketosis. These signs include:

1. **Bad breaths**

   When your body breaks down fat and protein as energy, there are by-products created that need to be eliminated. These by-products can be eliminated through sweat, poo, pee, and breadth. An excellent example of these by-products is acetone. Scott Keatley, R.D. of Keatley Medical Nutrition Therapy, states that "A little bit of acetone on the breath has a fruity smell, but a lot has a very distinct astringent smell that is quite unpleasant. He further stated that "This is a general sign that you're in ketosis and you're burning protein or fat as a source of energy." Many people experiencing this brush their teeth several times more than often or use sugar-free gums to solve the issue. It is important to note this: in case you are using gum or any other alternative asides from brushing, check the label for carbs. If you are not careful, you might increase your carb intake.

2. **Fatigue and tiredness**

   The period your body goes into ketosis, you will feel tired. This is because your body is not used to making use of fats and protein for energy and does not possess the average amount of carbs it will ordinarily use to burn energy. With time, your body will adjust accordingly.

3. Your appetite level will decrease

The rate at which you get hungry will be reduced. The reason for this is largely unclear. Keatley explained that there a couple of theories that shows why this happens. One of such could be that your new diet changes the bacteria in your guts. Another reason could be that your brain makes you think and feel less hungry.

4. You tend to have some disorders

When you eat keto foods, you are eating fat that is unusual to your body. Keatley further states that "Your body doesn't digest it properly, and the bacteria in your gut is not ready to break it down. This can lead to a temporary disorder. This should subside after a little bit, but you can always ease into a keto diet rather than jump all in to avoid these issues." After a while, it will stop. You must eat vegetables that are low in carbs and high in fibre.

5. You might experience weight loss in a week

Research has shown that ketogenic diets are highly effective for losing weight. The weight loss you will encounter might be both short-term weight loss and long-term weight loss. You can experience a fast weight loss in the first week. During this period, you will shed stored carbs and water.

6. Insomnia

When starting out keto foods, you may find it hard to sleep. Insomnia is widespread in most new ketogenic dieters. This also improves with time. In a matter of weeks, you might be sleeping better than the period before you started eating keto food.

History of Keto Diet

Before the term "Keto Diet" or "Ketogenic" was coined, the idea behind the diet plan already existed. Although these terms were not used until the twentieth century, a form of dieting called "fasting" was common for a long time. If you fast or do not eat anything for an extended period, your body will start to produce something called ketones or ketone bodies. Ketone bodies are produced when the body starts using stored fat to substitute for the lack of carbohydrates needed for energy production. The ancient man saw the importance of using fasting to achieve benefits in metabolic health, and this practice had been ongoing for centuries. There are several historical instances where fasting was used in the medical line. These instances include:

- Ancient Greek doctors used fasting to cure diseases.
- Hippocrates used fasting as a remedy for epilepsy and other health conditions. Fasting was also used for seizures/seizure control. Ketones and beta-hydroxybutyrate, a chemical produced from fasting, helped control seizures.
- In 1914, fasting was used to treat type 1 and type 2 diabetes.
- In 1922, an osteopath called Hugh Conklin made some adults and children with epilepsy fast for up 18 days at a stretch and sometimes up to 25 days, providing only limited liquids. He recorded a 50 per cent success rate in adults and 90 per cent in children.

It is safe to say, therefore, that the idea about the keto diet originated mostly from the usage of fasting to treat epilepsy and other disease conditions like myoclonic-astatic epilepsy, dravet syndrome, infantile spasms, and tuberous sclerosis.

Initially, the results achieved were remarkable. Yet, there was a problem. Since these fasts were temporary and only happened for a couple of days, it was discovered that many patients had their seizures once again when they resumed their previous diets. Other doctors started to practice these experiments and modified the fasts. They modified the fast by paying attention to ways to eliminate just starch and sugar alone, instead of eliminating all kinds of foods. This led to the birth of the classical ketogenic diet.

In 1921, Dr Russell Wilder from Mayo Clinic created the ketogenic diet. He used the diet as a treatment for extreme cases of intractable paediatric epilepsy in children. He noticed that some of his epileptic patients experienced a lesser number of seizures at certain times when their sugar level was low. This low blood sugar level was achieved by eating high fat and low carbohydrate diet. His keto diet plan calculated four parts fat for every one-part of protein and carb.

In the 1930s, however, this method was dropped. New and improved drugs for seizures were manufactured, and these anti convulsion drugs worked better. They were also easier to administer by doctors, while patients also found them easier and more effective to use. Thus, Dr Russell Wilder's idea was completely dropped and forgotten.

However, In the 1970s, the keto diet was revisited. During that period, there was a whole lot of emphasis placed on weight loss, and so consumers welcomed the idea of dieting. Despite this interest, the keto diet did not receive an instant welcome back, rather there were series of events that led to its revival. Here is a summary of the events:

- In 1972, a popular cardiologist called Dr Atkins released a book titled *the Diet Revolution*. He talked about low-carb dieting for weight loss and a good heart condition. Before this time, he had been researching weight loss and dieting. This was a huge steppingstone for a food diet that involves high fat and low carb.

- In 1977, another book about dieting was released. This time it was written by the physician and scientist, Dr Phinney. Before this period, he had spent his whole life on nutrition. The book he released was titled "The Last Chance Diet". The focus of the book was on the fat and protein diet drink. This didn't materialize as the drink he made was bad and did not contain important minerals. It also led to illnesses among people, and in some cases, caused death.

- Dr Phinney, however, created a new program in 1988. This time the program was called "The Optifast Diet. It was a nutritional program which was still focused on the fat and protein drinks he made. These drinks were an update from the previous one, and the program was endorsed by Oprah.

- The NBC aired a show that put a child on display after he was saved from epilepsy via Keto methods. This opened some more inquiry and prevalence for the Keto diet.

- Dr Atkins released an update on his previous book published in 1992, which was titled *Dr Atkins New Diet Revolution*. This book influenced other doctors in writing their own books on similar topics.

- In 1996, the story of an epileptic boy that got better through a keto diet plan was adapted into a movie (this was the boy that was featured by the NBC in 1990). This revived interests in ketogenic diet plans and their benefits.

- The early 2000s saw the rediscovery of the Atkins Diet. Also, the low-carb movement began gaining popularity.

- In 2013, a study was published in *Science* magazine showing the anti-ageing and health benefits of a ketogenic diet.
- Currently, the keto diet is immensely popular among people on a weight loss journey.

Importance and Benefits of Keto Diet

Doing a ketogenic diet has a couple of benefits. These benefits include:

1. Keto diet assists in losing weight. One of the main purpose people switch to this diet plan is to lose weight. It does this by boosting metabolism and reducing appetite. When your body lacks carbs that should have been converted to glucose, the body burns fats instead. Using fat as your main source of energy will make you stable and satiated. Foods eaten in this diet plan also reduce hormones that initiate hunger.

2. The keto diet helps to reduce acne. One of the main causes of acne for some people is excess blood sugar. When these people switch diets and begin to eat low-carb food, they begin to experience changes in acne. The balance of gut bacteria will be altered, and blood sugar reduces drastically.

3. It improves heart conditions. The diet also helps heart health by reducing inflammation and lowering oxidative stress. Furthermore, the fact that it aids weight loss guarantees positive impacts on the heart.

4. It reduces the risk of some types of cancer. Studies have shown that a ketogenic diet could be linked to increasing the number of days a cancer patient has to live. It has also been helpful in reducing the growth of tumours.

Types Of Keto Diet

There are several types of Keto Diets plan. These plans will be listed and discussed below:

1. Standard Ketogenic Dieting (SKD)
2. Targeted Ketogenic Dieting (TKD)
3. Cyclical Ketogenic Dieting (CKD)
4. High Protein Ketogenic Dieting
5. Calorie-restricted Ketogenic Dieting

Standard Ketogenic Dieting (SKD)

This type of diet can be regarded as the true keto diet. It consists of extremely low carb, moderate protein, and high fat. Typically, the diet contains 70 to 75 percent fat, 20 percent protein, and about 5 to 10 percent carbs. In terms of grams per day, a standard keto diet would be:

- 20-50g of carbohydrate
- 40-60g of protein
- No set limit for fat. The fat that will be taken provides most calories that would be needed. No limit is set because the energy requirements of people vary significantly.

If the main reason for taking up the keto diet is to lose weight, then the standard keto diet is a good place to start. Ketogenic diets should include a good intake of vegetables, particularly non-starchy vegetables, as these are exceptionally low in carbohydrates. Standard ketogenic diets have consistently recorded success in helping people to lose weight, improve their blood glucose level, control, and improve heart health.

Targeted Ketogenic Dieting (TKD)

Targeted Ketogenic Diet gives keto dieters the liberty to eat small carb-containing meals before or after they exercise. If you work out and follow the Standard Ketogenic Diet, you may discover that you would not have enough energy to work out. It is based on the concept that carbohydrates consumed before or after an exercise will be processed much more efficiently, as the muscles will demand energy increase because one is active.

You can add about 30 to 40 grams of carbs to your meal before or after your workout session. You should, however, note that you will need to cut back on the number of grams of fat you take for that day. When you do not have to exercise, you should stick to the Standard Ketogenic Diet.

Cyclical Ketogenic Dieting (CKD)

The Cyclical Ketogenic Dieting is also known as carb backloading or cycle keto diet. The concept behind this type of ketogenic dieting is to involve days in which you take in more carbs. For example, you can choose to follow the Standard Ketogenic Dieting strictly from Monday to Friday and then eat a high carb-filled diet on Saturdays and Sundays.

High Protein Ketogenic Dieting

This is like the Standard Ketogenic Dieting. The difference between the two dieting plans is that the High Protein Ketogenic Dieting contains more protein. The ratio is usually 35 per cent protein, 60 per cent fat, and 5 per cent carbs. This type of diet is also helpful for weight loss.

Calorie-Restricted Ketogenic Diet

A calorie-restricted ketogenic diet is almost like a standard ketogenic diet. The difference between both is that in a Calorie-restricted ketogenic diet, the calories are restricted to a specific amount. Research has, however, shown that both ketogenic diets are helpful in losing weight.

Keto Recipes

We have highlighted a couple of Keto recipes for different times of the day that will help you achieve all the benefits of a Keto diet. These recipes usually involve the use of specific ingredients for certain food items and the exclusion of other ingredients that are usually a part of food items.

Some of the foods that have been accepted for a standard keto diet include:
- Dairy products like yoghurt, cheese products, as well as milk.
- Protein: found in shellfish, pork, poultry, fish, beef, eggs, and soybeans.
- Seeds such as almonds and pumpkin seeds.
- Nuts such as walnuts, pecans, hazelnuts.
- Animal fats gotten from salmon and sardines.
- Plant based fats from an olive.
- Fruits like coconut, berries, avocado, and rhubarb.
- Starch-free vegetables like cauliflower, cabbage, and broccoli.

At the advent of the keto diet, physicians placed emphasis on taking exact measurements to achieve optimum results. This meant that food was studied and measured to the minutest details to ensure maximum result.

Keto Breakfast Recipes

KETO CEREAL

Makes 3 servings
Setting: low | Prep time: 10 minutes | Cook time: 35 mins

PER SERVING
Carbs: 36g | Protein: 29.9g | Fibre: 21g | Fat: 128.8g |
Kcal: 1076

INGREDIENTS

- 110g chopped almonds
- 120g chopped walnuts
- 85g unsweetened coconut flakes
- 150g sesame seeds
- 10g flax seeds
- 10g chia seeds
- 5g ground clove
- 15g ground cinnamon
- 15g pure vanilla extract
- 10g kosher salt
- 1 large egg white
- 1 cup of melted coconut oil

INSTRUCTIONS

1. Warm-up the oven to 180° Celsius. After this, grease a baking sheet with cooking spray.
2. Go ahead to mix almonds, walnuts, coconut flakes, and sesame seeds, flax seeds, and chia seeds in a large bowl. After doing that, ensure you stir in cloves, vanilla, salt, and cinnamon.
3. Beat egg white, stir into granola after it becomes foamy.
4. Add coconut oil and stir until all is well coated.

5. Pour onto the prepared baking sheet and spread it into an even layer. Bake until it is golden (usually about 25 minutes), gently stirring halfway through. Let cool completely.

You can use pistachios, pecans, or pumpkin seeds instead of almonds and walnuts. To sweeten the cereal, you can also add in some keto-friendly sweeteners. You can also decide to keep the granola stored in an air-tight container to keep it under room temperature.

KETO PANCAKE

Makes 3 servings
Setting: low | Prep time: 5 minutes | Cook time: 15 mins

PER SERVING
Carbs: 5.8g | Protein: 21.2g | Fibre: 0.5g | Fat: 99.7g | Kcal: 699

INGREDIENTS

- 50g almond flour
- 470g cream cheese, softened
- 4 large eggs
- 1 teaspoon lemon zest

INSTRUCTIONS

1. Mix and whisk the almond flour, cream cheese, eggs, and lemon zest together until smooth. This can be done in any size of a bowl depending on the quantity you would like to make.
2. Melt butter on the pan you choose to use (preferably a non-stick pan).
3. Pour the quantity of batter you wish to have per pancake on the pan.
4. Cook until it looks golden. Flip to the other side after two minutes.
5. Once you have cooked all the batter, you can transfer to any plate desired.
6. You can decide to add syrups.

KETO CLOUD BREAD

Makes 3 servings
Setting: low | Prep time: 5 minutes | Cook time: 15 mins

PER SERVING
Carbs: 13.2g | Protein: 7.7g | Fibre: 0g | Fat: 17.0g |
Kcal: 187

INGREDIENTS

- 3 large eggs, at room temperature
- 60g cream of tartar
- pinch of kosher salt
- 55g cream cheese, softened

INSTRUCTIONS

1. Warm-up the oven to 150° Celsius and line a large baking sheet with parchment paper.
2. Use two medium-sized bowls to separate the egg white from the yolk of the egg.
3. Add cream of tartar and salt to egg whites. Then use a hand mixer to beat the mixture for 2 to 3 minutes until stiff peaks.
4. Add cream cheese to egg yolks. Use the hand mixer again to mix.
5. Gently fold egg yolk and cream cheese mixture into egg whites.
6. Divide mixture into 3 mounds on the prepared baking sheet, spacing them about 4" apart. Bake until golden, 25 to 30 minutes.
7. Immediately sprinkle each piece of bread with cheese and bake for 2 to 3 minutes more till it is melty.
8. Let cool slightly.

HAM EGG & CHEESE ROLL-UPS

Makes 8 servings
Setting: medium | Prep time: 15 minutes | Cook time: 35 minutes

PER SERVING
Carbs: 7.1g | Protein: 31g | Fibre: 1.6g | Fat: 18.6g |
Kcal: 321

INGREDIENTS

- 10 large eggs
- 20g garlic powder
- kosher salt
- freshly ground black pepper
- 30g butter
- 350g shredded cheddar
- 30g baby spinach
- 220g tinned tomatoes
- 20 slices of ham

INSTRUCTIONS

1. Heat the grill.
2. Break the eggs into a large bowl. Whisk the eggs with garlic powder and add salt and pepper.
3. In a large non-stick frying pan over medium heat, melt butter.
4. Add eggs and scramble, occasionally stirring for about 3 minutes.
5. Stir in cheddar until it has melted.
6. After, stir in baby spinach and tomatoes until combined.

7. Place two slices of ham on a flat board. Add a spoon of the scrambled eggs and roll-up. Do this for the remaining ham and eggs.
8. Place the roll-ups in a shallow baking dish.
9. Boil for about 5 minutes until the ham is crispy.

AVOCADO EGG BOATS

Makes 7 servings
Setting: low | Prep time: 10 minutes | Cook time: 40 minutes

PER SERVING
Carbs: 5.3g | Protein: 7.7g | Fibre: 3.9g | Fat: 17.4g |
Kcal: 202

INGREDIENTS

- 2 ripe avocados
- 4 large eggs
- kosher salt
- freshly ground black pepper
- 3 slices of bacon
- freshly chopped chives for dressing

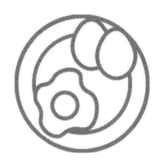

INSTRUCTIONS

1. Heat the oven up to 180° Celsius.
2. Out of each half of avocado, scoop a tablespoon worth of avocado; discard or reserve for another use.
3. Place hollowed avocados in a baking dish, then crack eggs into a bowl, one at a time. Using a spoon, transfer one yolk to each avocado half, then spoon in as much egg white as you can fit without spilling over.
4. Add salt and pepper as seasoning and bake for 20 to 25 minutes until whites are set, and yolks are no longer runny. (Cover with foil if avocados start getting brown.)
5. Meanwhile, in a large skillet over medium heat, cook bacon until crisp, 8 minutes, then transfer to a paper towel-lined plate and chop.
6. Top avocados with bacon and chives before serving.

LOW-CARB BREAKFAST HASH

Makes 6 servings
Setting: medium | Prep time: 10 minutes | Cook time: 50 minutes

PER SERVING
Carbs: 11g | Protein: 15g | Fibre: 4g | Fat: 13g |
Kcal: 220

INGREDIENTS

- 6 slices of bacon, cut into 1" pieces
- 1 chopped onion
- 1 chopped red bell pepper
- 1 chopped large head of cauliflower
- kosher salt
- freshly ground black pepper
- ½ teaspoon smoked paprika
- 50ml water
- 2 cloves of garlic, sliced
- 2 finely chopped chives
- 4 eggs
- 235g shredded cheddar cheese

INSTRUCTIONS

1. Fry bacon until it gets crispy using a large non-stick skillet and medium heat; ensure that you fry bacon until crispy. After this, turn off the heat and transfer the bacon to a paper plate (tower-lined). Remove any black pieces of bacon and keep a larger percentage of bacon fat in the skillet.

2. Add bell pepper and cauliflower to the skillet. Cook and occasionally stir till the vegetables begin to get soft and get golden. Use salt, paprika and pepper as seasoning.

3. Add 2 tablespoons of water, then cover the skillet. Cook until the cauliflower is tender, and the water has evaporated (for about 5 minutes). (If all the water evaporates before the cauliflower is tender, add more water to the skillet and cover for a couple of minutes more.)
4. Take off the lid, then stir in the garlic and chives, and cook until the garlic is fragrant for about 30 seconds.
5. Make four holes in the hash to show the bottom of the skillet using a wooden spoon.
6. Crack an egg into each hole and season each egg with salt and pepper. Sprinkle cheese and cooked bacon bits over the entire skillet.
7. Replace lid and cook until eggs are cooked to your liking, about 5 minutes for a runny egg. Serve warm.

BACON WEAVE BREAKFAST TACOS

Makes 4 servings
Setting: medium | Prep time: 10 minutes | Cook time: 60 minutes

PER SERVING
Carbs: 4g | Protein: 24g | Fibre: 2g | Fat: 31g |
Kcal: 390

INGREDIENTS

- 16 slices of bacon
- black pepper (freshly ground)
- 6 large eggs
- 15ml whole milk
- 18g butter
- kosher salt
- 2g chopped chives
- 90g shredded monterey jack
- 150g of sliced avocado
- hot sauce, for serving

INSTRUCTIONS

1. Make bacon taco shells: heat the oven to about 200° Celsius, then line a big, rimmed baking sheet with foil. At a corner, make a bacon weave with 8 halves of bacon each, creating a square. Repeat to make the next three weaves. Add pepper seasoning. To ensure the bacon is flat, place an inverted baking rack on top.

2. Bake Bacon until it is crisp (take about 30-35 minutes). Working quickly, trim each square with a paring knife or kitchen shears to make a round shape.

3. Meanwhile, make scrambled eggs: In a medium bowl, whisk together eggs with milk until well incorporated.

4. Melt butter over medium-low heat in a non-stick skillet. Pour in the egg mixture. Gently move the eggs around with a spatula, creating large curds when the eggs are almost cooked to your liking, season with salt and pepper. Fold in chives and remove from heat.

5. Assemble tacos: On a serving platter, top the bacon taco shells with scrambled eggs. Sprinkle each with cheese, nestled in a few slices of avocado, and top with hot sauce.

CAULIFLOWER TOAST

Makes 6 servings
Setting: medium | Prep time: 15 minutes | Cook time: 45 minutes

PER SERVING
Carbs: 5g | Protein: 5g | Fibre: 2g | Fat: 4g |
Kcal: 80

INGREDIENTS

- 1 medium head cauliflower
- 1 large egg
- 110g shredded cheddar
- 1 ½ teaspoon garlic powder
- kosher salt
- freshly ground black pepper

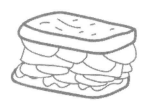

INSTRUCTIONS

1. Heat the oven to about 220° Celsius, then line a baking sheet with some parchment paper. Grate cauliflower finely, then transfer to a big container. For 8 minutes, microwave at a high temperature. Drain completely with paper towels or a cheesecloth until the mixture is dry.
2. Add egg, cheddar, and garlic powder to the cauliflower bowl and season with salt and pepper. Mix until combined.
3. Form cauliflower into toast shapes on a prepared baking sheet and bake until golden for about 18 minutes.
4. Move to a plate and add desired toppings like mashed avocado, a fried egg, or bacon, lettuce, and tomato.

Keto Lunch Recipes

KETO PROSCIUTTO MANCHEGO GRILLED SALAD

Makes 2 servings
Setting: low | Prep time: 5 minutes | Cook time: 15 minutes

PER SERVING
Carbs: 10.2g | Protein: 24.1g | Fibre: 5.4g | Fat: 56.8g |
Kcal: 642

INGREDIENTS

- 450g romaine lettuce
- 12 teaspoons olive oil, divided
- 170g prosciutto
- 240g manchego cheese
- 1/2 cup lemon juice
- 28g mayonnaise
- salt and pepper to taste

INSTRUCTIONS

1. Measure all the ingredients.
2. Preheat the grill at low heat temperature for about 20 minutes.
3. Divide half the head of the lettuce into two. Brush with half olive oil on both sides of the lettuce.
4. Put lettuce on the grill. Grill on the two sides for a couple of minutes and keep the grill lid open. Grill until the outer part is roasted.
5. Peel the cheese of manchego with a vegetable cutter or sharp knife. Cut the vegetable and the prosciutto into tiny bits.

6. Mix the bits of salad with remaining olive oil, mayonnaise, and lemon juice in a bowl. Toss to combine. Stir to mix properly.
7. Add the salad with the prosciutto and manchego.
8. Garnish with pepper and salt.
9. Serve.

KETO CREAMY CHICKEN SOUP

Makes 6 servings
Setting: low | Prep time: 10 minutes | Cook time: 30 minutes

PER SERVING
Carbs: 7.3g | Protein: 5.5g | Fibre: 2.3g | Fat: 14g |
Kcal: 170

INGREDIENTS

- 2 liters of filtered water
- 1 full chicken
- 400g cubed fresh pumpkin
- 1 lime juice
- 2 medium zucchinis
- 30g thinly sliced fresh parsley
- 1/2 cup thinly sliced fresh cilantro
- 1 ½ teaspoon ground turmeric
- 1 cup coconut cream
- 2 teaspoons apple cider vinegar
- 10g finely chopped ginger
- 2 teaspoons salt
- 2 shallots (optional)
- 4 cloves of garlic (optional)
- 1 teaspoon chili flakes (optional)
- black pepper, to taste

INSTRUCTIONS

1. Cover the chicken in a slow cooker with water and apple cider vinegar.
2. Cook for about 4 hours in a pot or slow cooker over low heat till the chicken is tender.

3. Remove the chicken from the pot with caution and put aside. Strain the bone or skin fragments and set aside the rest of the stock. Return the stock to the pot and stir in the pumpkin, zucchini, and ginger. Allow Simmer for about 15 minutes on low pressure. Cook for an extra 15 minutes, or until the pumpkin and zucchini are tender.

4. When the vegetables are frying, cut the meat from the chicken, and set it aside.

5. When the pumpkin has softened, whisk in the parsley, cilantro, shallots, lime juice, coconut milk, and chicken to cook up.

6. Taste the mixture and add the salt, lime juice, and spices to your taste.

7. Serve promptly, garnished with additional new herbs.

KETO BAGEL RECIPE

Makes 6 servings
Setting: medium | Prep time: 5 minutes | Cook time: 25 minutes

PER SERVING
Carbs: 19g | Protein: 19g | Fibre: 12g | Fat: 56g |
Kcal: 529

INGREDIENTS

- 120g almond flour
- 28g coconut flour
- 7g psyllium husk powder
- 2g baking powder
- 3g garlic powder
- pinch salt
- 2 medium eggs
- 10ml white wine vinegar
- 38ml melted ghee
- 15ml olive oil
- 5g sesame seeds

INSTRUCTIONS

1. Preheat the oven.
2. In a mixing cup, whisk together the coconut flour, almond flour, psyllium husk powder, baking powder, and salt.
3. Whisk together the eggs and vinegar in a separate dish. Slowly drizzle in the molten ghee (which should not be boiling) and whisk properly.

4. Combine the wet and dry mixtures with a wooden spoon. Enable to stay for 2-3 minutes.
5. Divide the mixture into equal-sized parts. Shape the mixture into a circular shape with your hands and put it on a tray lined with parchment paper. To make the middle hole, use a small spoon or apple corer.

CREAMY AVOCADO CUCUMBER GAZPACHO

Makes 6 servings
Setting: medium | Prep time: 15 minutes | Cook time: 15 minutes

PER SERVING
Carbs: 8.43g | Protein: 1.6g | Fibre: 2.3g | Fat: 14g |
Kcal: 95

INGREDIENTS

- 2 medium cucumbers peeled, seeded, and chopped
- 220g sliced avocados
- 1 cup of water
- 1 jalapeno seeded and chopped
- 6g loosely packed cilantro or basil leaves
- 230g apple cider vinegar
- 2 garlic cloves
- 1 teaspoon of salt
- 3/4 teaspoon of pepper

INSTRUCTIONS

1. Combine the cucumbers, avocado, jalapeno, cilantro, vinegar, garlic, salt, and pepper in a food processor. Blend until smooth.
2. Blend with water, then apply more if needed to thin it out.
3. Season with salt and pepper to taste.

KETO TACO CUPS

Makes 12 servings
Setting: medium | Prep time: 10 minutes | Cook time: 30 minutes

PER SERVING
Carbs: 2g | Protein: 25g | Fibre: 0g | Fat: 21g |
Kcal: 300

INGREDIENTS

- 160g shredded cheddar
- 3 teaspoons extra-virgin olive oil
- 1 small onion, chopped
- 3 sliced garlic cloves
- 450g ground beef
- ½ teaspoon chilli powder
- ½ teaspoon ground cumin
- ½ teaspoon paprika
- kosher salt
- black pepper (freshly ground)
- sour cream, for serving
- diced avocado for serving
- freshly chopped cilantro, for serving
- chopped tomatoes for serving

INSTRUCTIONS

1. Heat the oven to 190° Celsius and then line a large baking sheet with parchment paper.
2. Set about 2 tablespoons cheddar. Bake until bubbly and edges begin to turn golden (about 6 minutes). Let cool on the baking sheet for a minute.

3. Meanwhile, grease the bottom of a muffin tin with cooking spray, then carefully pick up melted cheese slices and place them on the bottom of the muffin tin. Fit with another muffin tin and allow cool for ten minutes. Where you lack a second muffin tin, employ your hands to mould the cheese around the inverted tin.

4. Heat oil in a large skillet, using heat at a medium.

5. Add onion and cook; occasionally stir till it softens (will take about 5 minutes).

6. Stir in garlic, add ground beef, and break up the meat with a wooden spoon. Cook till beef is no longer pink (should take 6 minutes) and drain the fat.

7. Return meat to the skillet and use chilli powder, cumin, pepper, paprika, and salt.

8. Transfer cheese cups to a serving platter. Fill with cooked ground beef and top with sour cream, avocado, cilantro, and tomatoes.

EGG ROLL BOWLS

Makes 4 servings
Setting: medium | Prep time: 10 minutes | Cook time: 35 minutes

PER SERVING
Carbs: 11g | Protein: 22g | Fibre: 3g | Fat: 32g |
Kcal: 420

INGREDIENTS

- 1 tablespoon vegetable oil
- 1 garlic clove, sliced
- 5g sliced fresh ginger
- 450g ground pork
- 1 tablespoon sesame oil
- 1/2 onion, thinly sliced
- 110g shredded carrot
- 250g green cabbage, thinly sliced
- ½ cup of soy sauce
- 15g Sriracha
- kosher salt
- 1 green onion, thinly sliced
- 9g toasted sesame seeds

INSTRUCTIONS

1. Heat vegetable oil over medium heat. To make it fragrant, add garlic and ginger, then cook (will take a minute).
2. Add pork and cook, occasionally stirring, till meat is golden in parts and cooked through, 8 to 10 minutes, breaking meat into small pieces with a spatula or spoon.
3. Move pork to one side and add sesame oil.

4. Add onion, carrot, and cabbage. Stir to combine with meat and add soy sauce and Sriracha. Cook until cabbage is tender, 5 to 8 minutes. Season to taste with salt.

5. Transfer mixture to a serving dish and garnish with green onions and sesame seeds. Serve.

NO-BREAD ITALIAN SUBS

Makes 6 servings
Setting: medium | Prep time: 15 minutes | Cook time: 15 minutes

PER SERVING
Carbs: 3g | Protein: 16g | Fibre: 0g | Fat: 34g |
Kcal: 390

INGREDIENTS

- 110g mayonnaise
- 2 tablespoons red wine vinegar
- 1 tablespoon extra-virgin olive oil
- 1 small garlic clove, grated
- 14g Italian seasoning
- 6 slices of ham
- 12 slices of salami
- 12 slices of pepperoni
- 6 slices provolone
- 50g shredded romaine
- 150g roasted red peppers

INSTRUCTIONS

1. Make Italian dressing that is creamy: In a small-sized bowl, whisk mayonnaise together with oil, garlic, and Italian seasoning till emulsified.
2. Gather sandwiches: Layer a slice of ham, two pieces of salami, two slices of pepperoni, and a slice of provolone.
3. Add a handful of romaine and a few roasted red peppers in the middle. Drizzle with creamy Italian dressing, then roll up and serve. Repeat with the remaining ingredients until you have 6 roll-ups.

Keto Dinner Recipes

GARLICKY LEMON MAHI-MAHI

Makes 4 servings
Setting: medium | Prep time: 10 minutes | Cook time: 30 mins

PER SERVING
Carbs: 0g | Protein: 21g | Fibre: 0g | Fat: 13g |
Kcal: 200

INGREDIENTS

- 14g butter, divided
- 2 tablespoons olive oil (extra-virgin)
- black pepper (freshly ground)
- 450g asparagus
- kosher salt
- 3 sliced cloves of garlic,
- 110g mahi-mahi fillets
- ¼ tablespoon crushed red pepper flakes
- 1 peeled and chopped lemon
- 1 lemon (zest and Juice)
- 4g freshly chopped parsley; you might need extra for garnish

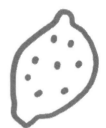

INSTRUCTIONS

1. In a big skillet at medium heat, melt a tablespoon each of butter and olive oil.
2. Add mahi-mahi and use salt and pepper as seasonings. Cook until golden, 4 to 5 minutes per side. Transfer to a plate.
3. Add the remaining oil to the skillet. Add asparagus and then cook till it is tender (2-4 minutes).

4. Add salt and pepper as seasonings, and transfer to a plate.
5. To skillet, add the remaining butter.
6. Once melted, add garlic and red pepper flakes, and cook until fragrant (about 1 minute), then stir in lemon, zest, juice, and parsley. Remove from heat, then return mahi-mahi and asparagus to skillet and spoon over the sauce.
7. Garnish with more parsley before serving.

CAULIFLOWER FRIED RICE

Makes 4 servings
Setting: medium | Prep time: 5 minutes | Cook time: 20 minutes

PER SERVING
Carbs: 17.3g | Protein: 5g | Fibre: 5.5g | Fat: 0.4g |
Kcal: 108

INGREDIENTS

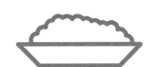

- 1 head cauliflower to be cut into florets
- 2 tablespoons of vegetable oil
- 1 bunch of scallion, ensure that they are thinly sliced
- 3 minced garlic cloves
- 1 tablespoon of fresh ginger (minced)
- 2 carrots (peeled and diced)
- 2 diced celery stalks
- 1 diced red bell pepper
- 1 cup of frozen peas
- 2 tablespoons of rice vinegar
- 3 tablespoons of soy sauce
- 2 teaspoons of sriracha for taste

INSTRUCTIONS

1. In making the fried rice: using the bowl of a food processor, pulse your cauliflower till the mixture resembles rice (should take 2-3 minutes). Then set aside.

2. Heat oil in a large skillet at medium heat. Add garlic, ginger, scallions then stir-fry till it is fragrant (should take a minute).

3. Add red bell pepper, celery and carrots, and fry till the vegetables are very tender (takes about 9-11 minutes).

4. Add the cauliflower rice and fry till it turns golden (should take 3-5 minutes). Add in the frozen peas, stir, and toss well to ensure that they combine.

5. Add soy sauce, sriracha, and rice vinegar and then toss to combine. Set aside after this.

6. In making the garnishes: Heat oil at medium heat in a medium skillet. Crack eggs into the pan, and keep cooking till the yolks are runny, but the whites are set (should take 3-4 minutes). Use salt and pepper as seasonings.

7. In serving, divide the cauliflower rice into four plates and add fried eggs as a topping for each one. Garnish each plate with 1 tablespoon scallions, 1 teaspoon sesame seeds, and 1 tablespoon cilantro. Serve immediately.

PHILLY CHEESESTEAK LETTUCE WRAPS

Makes 4 servings
Setting: medium | Prep time: 10 minutes | Cook time: 30 minutes

PER SERVING
Carbs: 7g | Protein: 31g | Fibre: 2g | Fat: 3g |
Kcal: 370

INGREDIENTS

- 2 tablespoons of vegetable oil
- 1 chopped large onion
- 2 large bell peppers
- kosher salt
- 2g dried oregano
- grounded black pepper (fresh)
- 450g skirt steak
- 110g provolone, shred it
- 8 big butterhead lettuce leaves
- 4g freshly chopped parsley

INSTRUCTIONS

1. Heat a tablespoon of oil, making use of a big skillet and medium heat. Include onion and some bell peppers, using salt, pepper, and oregano as seasoning. Cook, ensuring that you stir often and till the vegetables become tender (should take 10 minutes). Heat the leftover oil in the skillet after removing onions and pepper from it.
2. Add a steak to a layer, then season with pepper and salt. Cook till the steak has become seared on a part, then flip for it to sear on the other side (it should take 4 minutes in total).

3. Add onion mixture to the skillet and then combine by tossing. On the steak, sprinkle provolone, after which cover with lid (make it tight-fitting). Cook cheese until it melts; this should take a minute. You can then remove from heat.

4. Place lettuce on a serving platter. Then, spread the steak mixture on each arranged piece of lettuce. Garnish everything with parsley, then serve warm.

CREAMY TUSCAN CHICKEN

Makes 4 servings
Setting: medium | Prep time: 5 minutes | Cook time: 40 minutes

PER SERVING
Carbs: 5g | Protein: 29g | Fibre: 1g | Fat: 28g |
Kcal: 380

INGREDIENTS

- 3 teaspoons of extra-virgin olive oil
- 4 chicken breasts
- kosher salt
- freshly ground black pepper
- 1g dried oregano
- 42g butter
- 9g cloves of garlic
- 220g cherry tomatoes, halved
- 90g baby spinach
- 120g heavy cream
- 25g freshly grated Parmesan
- lemon wedges, for serving

INSTRUCTIONS

1. Remove the skin of the chicken breast, as well as bones.
2. In a skillet, over medium heat, heat oil.
3. Add chicken and season with salt, pepper, and oregano. Cook until golden and no longer pink, (8 minutes per side). Remove from skillet and set aside.
4. In the same skillet over medium heat, melt butter.
5. For a minute, stir in garlic and cook until it is fragrant. Add cherry tomatoes and season with salt and pepper.

6. Cook until tomatoes are beginning to burst, then add spinach and cook until spinach is beginning to wilt.

7. Stir in heavy cream and parmesan and bring mixture to a simmer. Reduce heat to low and simmer until sauce is slightly reduced (should take about 3 minutes). Return chicken to skillet and cook until heated through for 5 to 7 minutes.

8. Serve with lemon wedges.

GARLICKY SHRIMP ZUCCHINI PASTA

Makes 4 servings
Setting: medium | Prep time: 5 minutes | Cook time: 40 minutes

PER SERVING
Carbs: 5g | Protein: 24g | Fibre: 3g | Fat: 30g |
Kcal:410

INGREDIENTS

- 40g butter
- 1 large shrimp, peeled and deveined
- kosher salt
- black pepper (freshly ground)
- 3 sliced cloves of garlic
- 20g heavy cream
- 45g grated Parmesan
- 155g halved cherry tomatoes
- 12g chopped parsley
- 50g large zucchini, spiralled (or about 4 cups zoodles)

INSTRUCTIONS

1. Melt a tablespoon of butter using a large skillet. Add shrimp and use salt and pepper to season it. Cook till shrimp is opaque and pink (takes about 2 minutes). Move shrimp to a plate but keep juices in the skillet.

2. Melt leftover butter in a skillet and stir in garlic. Cook till it is fragrant (should take a minute), then whisk in heavy cream. Bring to simmer, and stir in parsley, tomatoes, and parmesan. Simmer until tomatoes soften and mixture thickens slightly for 3 minutes.

3. Return shrimp to skillet and add zucchini noodles. Toss to combine and serve immediately.

KETO HOT DOGS

Makes 6 servings
Setting: medium | Prep time: 15 minutes | Cook time: 25 minutes

PER SERVING
Carbs: 13g | Protein: 28g | Fibre: 5g | Fat: 49g |
Kcal: 590

INGREDIENTS

- 200g shredded mozzarella
- 110g cream cheese
- 2 large eggs, beaten
- 240g almond flour
- 2 teaspoons of baking powder
- 1 teaspoon of kosher salt
- 8 hot dogs
- 60g melted butter
- 1 tablespoon of garlic powder
- 4g freshly chopped parsley
- mustard, for serving

INSTRUCTIONS

1. Heat up the oven to 200° Celsius and line a baking sheet (make use of parchment paper).
2. In a big-sized microwave-safe bowl, melt together cream cheese and mozzarella.
3. Add eggs and stir to combine, then add almond flour, baking powder, and salt.
4. Divide dough into 4 balls, then shape each ball into long ropes.

5. Wrap a rope around each hot dog.
6. Whisk garlic, butter, parsley, and powder in a small bowl together.
7. Brush garlic butter over each hot dog, then bake until golden, 1o-15 minutes.
8. Serve with mustard.

CHEESE TACO SHELLS

Makes 4 servings
Setting: medium | Prep time: 20 minutes | Cook time: 30 minutes

PER SERVING
Carbs: 4g | Protein: 39g | Fibre: 1g | Fat: 28g |
Kcal: 430

INGREDIENTS

- 170g shredded cheddar
- freshly ground black pepper
- 1 tablespoon of vegetable oil
- 1 white onion, chopped
- 450g ground beef
- ½ teaspoon of taco seasoning
- shredded lettuce for serving
- chopped tomatoes for serving
- hot sauce, for serving

INSTRUCTIONS

1. Heat the oven up to 190° Celsius degrees.
2. Line a baking sheet (use parchment paper) and with cooking spray.
3. Put cheddar on the baking sheet and use pepper as seasoning.
4. Bake till cheese is melty and a little crispy (takes 5-7 minutes). Remove grease using paper towels.
5. Also, set up 4 stations of two upside-down glasses, as well as of a wooden spoon functioning as a bridge. Move cheese mounds to wooden spoons to form shells using a spatula.

6. Also, make taco meat and heat oil in a large skillet. Add onions, then cook for 5 minutes, and add ground beef and cook till it is no longer pink (should take 6 minutes more). Use taco seasoning to drain fat.

7. Assemble tacos: Place beef in shells and top with lettuce, tomatoes, and hot sauce.

Keto Dessert Recipes

CHEESY BAKED ASPARAGUS

Makes 6 servings
Setting: medium | Prep time: 10 minutes | Cook time: 30 minutes

PER SERVING
Carbs: 8g | Protein: 14g | Fibre: 3g | Fat: 19g |
Kcal: 250

INGREDIENTS

- 900g asparagus, stalks trimmed
- 180g heavy cream
- 3 cloves of garlic, sliced
- kosher salt
- black pepper (freshly ground)
- 90g freshly grated Parmesan
- 100g shredded mozzarella
- red pepper flakes, for garnish (optional)

INSTRUCTIONS

1. Heat the oven up to 200° Celsius.
2. Put asparagus in a 9"-x-13" baking dish and pour over some heavy cream, as well as scatter with garlic.
3. Add a great deal of salt and pepper, then sprinkle with parmesan, mozzarella, and red pepper flakes (if using).
4. Bake until cheese is golden and melty, and asparagus is tender, about 25 to 30 minutes, and serve.

KETO SUGAR-FREE CHEESECAKE

Makes 10 servings
Setting: medium | Prep time: 15 minutes | Cook time: 8 hours

PER SERVING
Carbs: 10g | Protein: 10g | Fibre: 3g | Fat: 47g |
Kcal: 500

INGREDIENTS

- 50g almond flour
- 58g coconut flour
- 18g shredded coconut
- 115g butter, melted
- 90g cream cheese, softened to room temperature
- 490g sour cream, at room temperature
- 6g stevia
- 10ml of vanilla (pure extract)
- 3 large eggs, at room temperature
- sliced strawberries for serving

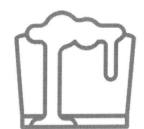

INSTRUCTIONS

1. Heat the oven to 150° Celsius.
2. Make the crust: Lubricate an 8" or 9" springform pan, and cover the bottom and edges using foil. In a bowl of medium size, mix butter, flour, and coconut. Press the crust to the bottom and up the sides of the pan that has been prepared. While you make the filling, place the pan in the fridge.

3. Preparing the filling- Beat Cream Cheese and Sour Cream together in a large bowl, then beat Vanilla and Stevia together. Include eggs one at a time and mix after each addition. Put the cheesecake in a deep roasting pan and set in the oven (use the middle rack).

4. Carefully pour enough boiling water into the roasting pan to come halfway up the sides of the springform pan. Bake for 1 hour- 1 hour 20 minutes, till there is a slight jiggle at the centre.

5. Turn off the oven; however, leave the cake within with the door opened to help it cool off (this should take only one hour).

6. Remove the foil from the pan, and take it away from the bathwater, then let chill in the fridge for at least five hours or overnight. Slice and garnish with strawberries.

KETO CHOCOLATE CHIP COOKIES

Makes 18 servings
Setting: medium | Prep time: 15 minutes | Cook time: 30 minutes

PER SERVING
Carbs: 8.1g | Protein: 1.7g | Fibre: 0g | Fat: 17.4g |
Kcal: 189

INGREDIENTS

- 2 large eggs
- 115g melted butter
- 480g heavy cream
- 10ml pure vanilla extract
- 265g almond flour
- 1.5g kosher salt
- 50g keto-friendly granulated sugar
- 120g dark chocolate chips
- cooking spray

INSTRUCTIONS

1. Heat the oven up to 180° Celsius.
2. Mix vanilla with butter and the egg using a large bowl. Add in the almond flour, salt, and Swerve.
3. Put the chocolate chips in the cookie batter.
4. Form the batter into 1" balls and arrange 3" apart on parchment-lined baking sheets.
5. Make the balls flat with the bottom of a glass that has been lightly lubricated with cooking spray.
6. Bake until the cookies are lightly golden (should take about 17-19 minutes).

KETO CHOCOLATE MUG CAKE

Makes 1 serving
Setting: low | Prep time: 5 minutes | Cook time: 5 minutes

PER SERVING
Carbs: 13g | Protein: 15g | Fibre: 7g | Fat: 44g |
Kcal: 470

INGREDIENTS

- 120g butter
- 25g almond flour
- 2 tablespoons of cocoa powder
- 1 large egg, beaten
- 20g keto-friendly chocolate chips
- 2 tablespoons granulated Swerve
- 115g baking powder
- pinch of kosher salt
- 60g whipped cream for serving

INSTRUCTIONS

1. Put butter in a microwave-safe mug, then heat till it is melted (about 30 seconds).
2. Include the rest of the ingredients and stir till they are fully combined (don't add whipped cream).
3. Cook for 45 seconds to 1 minute, or till the cake is set but still fudgy.
4. Top with whipped cream to serve.

KETO ICE-CREAM

Makes 12 servings
Setting: low | Prep time: 5 minutes | Cook time: 15 minutes

PER SERVING
Carbs: 7.5g | Protein: 10g | Fibre: 7g | Fat: 24.1g |
Kcal: 250

INGREDIENTS

- 2 cups of coconut milk
- 480g heavy cream
- 50g swerve sweetener (confectioner).
- 5ml pure vanilla extract
- a drop of kosher salt

INSTRUCTIONS

1. Using a fridge for about 3 hours, chill coconut milk.
2. Making whipped coconut: Get coconut cream into a large bowl and use a hand mixer to beat the cream until it is very creamy. You can then set aside.
3. To make the whipped cream: Using a separate bowl and a hand mixer, mix the heavy cream until soft peaks appear. You can then beat in vanilla and sweetener.
4. Place whipped coconut in whipped cream, then move the mix to a loaf pan.
5. Allow mixture to get frozen (should take 5 hours).

KETO HOT CHOCOLATE

Makes 6 serving
Setting: low | Prep time: 5 minutes | Cook time: 10 minutes

PER SERVING
Carbs: 3.4g | Protein: 0.7g | Fibre: 0.4g | Fat: 4g |
Kcal: 47

INGREDIENTS

- 2 tablespoons of unsweetened cocoa powder, plus more for garnish
- 10.5g keto-friendly sugar
- 1 ¼ cups of water
- 60g heavy cream
- 1ml pure vanilla extract
- whipped cream for serving

INSTRUCTIONS

1. Over medium heat and in a small saucepan, whisk together cocoa, swerve, and about 2 tablespoons water until smooth and dissolved.
2. Increase heat to medium, add remaining water and cream, and occasionally whisk until hot.
3. Stir in vanilla and pour into a mug.
4. Serve with whipped cream and a dusting of cocoa powder.

MAGIC KETO COOKIES

Makes 6 serving
Setting: low | Prep time: 10 minutes | Cook time: 35 minutes

PER SERVING
Carbs: 2g | Protein: 2g | Fibre: 1g | Fat: 13g |
Kcal: 130

INGREDIENTS

- 1/4 cup of coconut oil
- 40g butter
- 3 tablespoons of granulated swerve sweetener
- 3g kosher salt
- 4 large egg yolks
- 160g sugar-free dark chocolate chips
- 1 cup of coconut flakes
- 3/4 cup of roughly chopped walnuts

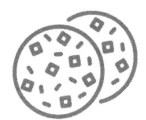

INSTRUCTIONS

1. Heat the oven to 180° Celsius.
2. Line a baking sheet using parchment paper.
3. Stir together coconut oil, butter, salt, sweetener, and egg yolks using a large bowl. Mix in chocolate chips, coconut, and walnuts.
4. Drop a spoonful of batter onto the prepared baking sheet and bake until golden for 15 minutes.

KETO FROSTY

Makes 4 serving
Setting: low | Prep time: 10 minutes | Cook time: 45 minutes

PER SERVING
Carbs: 4g | Protein: 2g | Fibre: 1g | Fat: 34g |
Kcal: 320

INGREDIENTS

- 360g heavy whipping cream
- 11g unsweetened cocoa powder
- 40g keto-friendly powdered sugar
  sweetener
- 5ml pure vanilla extract
- a pinch of kosher salt

INSTRUCTIONS

1. Combine cream, vanilla, sweetener, cocoa, and salt using a large bowl. Make use of a hand mixer or the whisk attachment of a stand mixer to beat the mixture until stiff peaks form. Scoop mixture into a Ziploc bag and freeze 30 to 35 minutes until just frozen.
2. Cut the tip off a corner of the Ziploc bag and pipe into serving dishes.

KETO BROWNIES

Makes 16 serving
Setting: low | Prep time: 15 minutes | Cook time: 1 hour 25 minutes

PER SERVING
Carbs: 11g | Protein: 7g | Fibre: 5g | Fat: 23g |
Kcal: 260

INGREDIENTS

- 4 large eggs
- 2 ripe avocados
- 115g melted butter
- 100g unsweetened peanut butter
- 2 teaspoons baking soda
- 80g keto-friendly granulated sugar (such as Swerve)
- 80g unsweetened cocoa powder
- 10ml pure vanilla extract
- 3g kosher salt
- flaky sea salt (optional)

INSTRUCTIONS

1. Get the oven 180° Celsius and line an 8"-x-8" square pan using parchment paper.
2. Blend all ingredients, except flaky sea salt, in a blender or food processor, ensure that you blend till smooth.
3. Move batter to prepared baking pan and smooth top with a spatula. Top with flaky sea salt (if desired).
4. Bake until brownies are soft but firm to touch, 25 to 30 minutes.
5. Let cool 25 to 30 minutes before slicing and serving.

KETO DOUBLE CHOCOLATE MUFFINS

Makes 12 serving
Setting: low | Prep time: 10 minutes | Cook time: 25 minutes

PER SERVING
Carbs: 7g | Protein: 7g | Fibre: 5g | Fat: 27g |
Kcal: 280

INGREDIENTS

- 190g almond flour
- 90g cocoa powder (unsweetened)
- 50g swerve sweetener
- 7g baking powder
- 6g kosher salt
- 225g butter (make it melted)
- 3 big eggs
- 5ml vanilla extract (pure)
- 160g chocolate chips

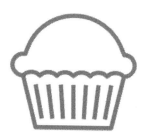

INSTRUCTIONS

1. Get the oven 180° Celsius and then line a muffin tin.
2. Using a big bowl, beat almond flour, swerve, cocoa powder, baking powder, and salt together. Add eggs, melted butter, vanilla and stir until combined.
3. Add chocolate chips by folding them in.
4. Share batter among muffin liners and bake till a toothpick put into the middle comes out clean. This should be done for 12 minutes.

COOKIE DOUGH KETO FAT BOMBS

Makes 12 serving
Setting: low | Prep time: 5 minutes | Cook time: 1 hour 5 minutes

PER SERVING
Carbs: 2g | Protein: 2g | Fibre: 1g | Fat: 7g |
Kcal: 280

INGREDIENTS

- 115g butter, softened
- 60g keto-friendly confectioners' sugar
- 2ml pure vanilla extract
- 3g kosher salt
- 192g almond flour
- 110g keto-friendly dark chocolate chips

INSTRUCTIONS

1. Beat butter till it is fluffy and light, using a hand mixer as well as a large bowl. Add sugar, vanilla, and salt and beat till they mix.
2. Slowly beat in almond flour till there is no dry spot, then fold in chocolate chips. Cover the bowl with plastic wrap and place it in the refrigerator to get it firm slightly (it takes about 15 to 20 minutes).
3. Using a small-sized cookie scoop, scoop dough into small balls.
4. Store in the refrigerator if planning to eat during the week or put in the freezer for up to 1 month.

KETO AVOCADO POPS

Makes 12 servings
Setting: low | Prep time: 5 minutes | Cook time: 6 hours 10 minutes

PER SERVING
Carbs: 52g | Protein: 1g | Fibre: 3g | Fat: 12g |
Kcal: 120

INGREDIENTS

- 3 ripe avocados
- ½ cup of lime juice
- 50g swerve or other sugar alternatives
- 4 teaspoons of coconut milk
- 1 tablespoon of coconut oil
- 160g keto-friendly chocolate

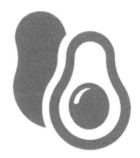

INSTRUCTIONS

1. Into a blender or food processor, mix avocados with lime juice, swerve, and coconut milk. Blend until smooth and pour into popsicle mould.
2. Freeze until firm (takes up to 6 hours or overnight).
3. In a medium bowl, combine chocolate chips and coconut oil. Microwave until melted, then let cool to room temperature.
4. Dunk frozen pops in chocolate and serve.

KETO CHOCOLATE TRUFFLES

Makes 15 servings
Setting: low | Prep time: 10 minutes | Cook time: 30 minutes

PER SERVING
Carbs: 2g | Protein: 1g | Fibre: 1g | Fat: 2g |
Kcal: 120

INGREDIENTS

- 160g dark chocolate chips, melted
- 1 medium avocado, mashed
- 5ml vanilla extract
- 1.5g kosher salt
- 30g cocoa powder

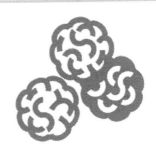

INSTRUCTIONS

1. Combine melted chocolate with salt, avocado, vanilla in a bowl of medium size. Stir together until smooth and fully combined—place in the refrigerator to firm up slightly (takes 15- 20 minutes).
2. When the chocolate mixture has stiffened, use a small-sized cookie scoop or small spoon to scoop approximately 1 tablespoon chocolate mixture.
3. Roll chocolate in the palm of your hand till it becomes round, then roll in cocoa powder.

CARROT CAKE KETO BALLS

Makes 16 servings
Setting: low | Prep time: 5 minutes | Cook time: 15 minutes

PER SERVING
Carbs: 6g | Protein: 2g | Fibre: 3g | Fat: 11g |
Kcal: 130

INGREDIENTS

- 25g cream cheese
- 80g coconut flour
- 6g stevia
- 2ml pure vanilla extract
- 2g cinnamon
- ¼ teaspoon of ground nutmeg
- 110g grated carrots
- 65g chopped pecans
- 100g coconut (shredded and unsweetened)

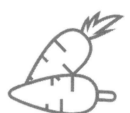

INSTRUCTIONS

1. Using a big bowl and a hand mixer, beat together stevia, vanilla, and cream cheese.
2. Add in pecans and carrots.
3. Serve after rolling into 16 balls and adding shredded coconut to each ball.

KETO FAT BOMBS

Makes 16 servings
Setting: low | Prep time: 5 minutes | Cook time: 30 minutes

PER SERVING
Carbs: 5g | Protein: 5g | Fibre: 1g | Fat: 28g |
Kcal: 290

INGREDIENTS

- 220g cream softened cheese
- 120g keto-friendly peanut butter
- ½ cup of coconut oil
- 1g kosher salt
- 80g keto-friendly dark chocolate chips

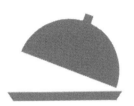

INSTRUCTIONS

1. Line a small baking sheet with parchment paper. In a bowl of medium- size, combine cream cheese, peanut butter, ¼ cup coconut oil, and salt.
2. Using a hand mixer, beat the mixture until fully combined, about 2 minutes. Place bowl in the freezer to firm up slightly for 10 to 15 minutes.
3. When the peanut butter mixture has hardened, use a small cookie scoop or spoon to create tablespoon-sized balls — place in refrigerator to harden, 5 minutes.
4. Make the chocolate drizzle: combine chocolate chips and remaining coconut oil in a microwave-safe bowl and microwave in 30-second intervals till fully melted. Drizzle over peanut butter balls and place them back in the refrigerator for them to harden for 5 minutes.
5. To store, keep covered in refrigerator.

KETO AVOCADO BROWNIES

Makes 7 servings
Setting: low | Prep time: 5 minutes | Cook time: 30 minutes

PER SERVING
Carbs: 9.78g | Protein: 4g | Fibre: 7g | Fat: 9g |
Kcal: 290

INGREDIENTS

- 250g avocado, mashed
- 1/2 teaspoon vanilla
- 30g cocoa powder
- 3 teaspoons coconut oil or butter, ghee, shortening, lard
- 2 eggs
- 80g chocolate chips, melted
- 90g blanched almond flour
- 1/4 teaspoon baking soda
- 5g baking powder
- 1/4 teaspoon salt
- 60g erythritol
- 6g stevia powder

INSTRUCTIONS

1. Heat the oven to 180° Celsius.
2. In a separate bowl, combine the dry ingredients and whisk them together.
3. Peel the avocados. Weigh or measure your avocados. Place in a food processor. Process until smooth.

4. Add each wet ingredient to the food processor (one-by-one), and process for some seconds till all the wet ingredients have been included in the food processor.
5. Add the dry ingredients to the food processor, then mix until combined.
6. Place a piece of parchment paper over a 30x20cm (12"x8") baking dish and pour the batter into it. Spoon evenly. Bake for 30 minutes, or till a toothpick inserted in the middle comes out half clean. The top ought to be soft when you touch it with your fingers.

Keto Side Dishes Recipes

CHEESY BRUSSELS SPROUT BAKE

Makes 6 servings
Setting: low | Prep time: 15 minutes | Cook time: 20 minutes

PER SERVING
Carbs: 13g | Protein: 13g | Fibre: 6g | Fat: 25g |
Kcal: 320

INGREDIENTS

- 5 slices of bacon
- 40g butter
- 2 small shallots, sliced
- 900g brussels sprouts, halved
- kosher salt
- 1g cayenne pepper
- 180g heavy cream
- 60g shredded sharp white cheddar
- 50g gruyère

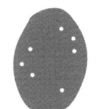

INSTRUCTIONS

1. Heat the oven to 190° Celsius. Cook bacon till crispy at medium heat in a large oven-safe skillet, should take about 8 minutes. Drain on a paper towel-lined plate and chop. Throw away bacon fat.
2. Melt butter with a skillet at medium heat. Add shallots and Brussels sprouts and use salt and cayenne as seasoning. Cook, occasionally stirring, till it is tender (takes about 10 minutes).
3. Remove from heat and drizzle with heavy cream, then top with both pieces of cheese and bacon.
4. Bake until cheese is bubbly (about 12-15 minutes). (If your cheese isn't golden, switch the oven to broil for 1 minute.)

CAULIFLOWER MAC AND CHEESE

Makes 6 servings
Setting: medium | Prep time: 15 minutes | Cook time: 30 minutes

PER SERVING
Carbs: 21.7g | Protein: 19g | Fibre: 3.8g | Fat: 19.5g |
Kcal: 331

INGREDIENTS

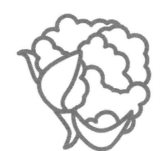

- 2 medium heads cauliflower, cut into florets
- 110g unsalted butter
- 60g flour
- 3 cups of milk
- 5g hot sauce, such as Flying Goose Hoi Sin Sauce
- 6g kosher salt
- 5g mustard powder
- freshly ground black pepper
- 240g shredded cheddar
- 200g mozzarella
- finely chopped chives for garnish

INSTRUCTIONS

1. In a pot of boiling water (make it large), scald cauliflower till it is tender (should take 5 to 7 minutes).
2. In a large saucepan, melt butter. Sprinkle over the flour and cook till slightly golden (takes 2-3 minutes). Add in milk and shake until combined. Use mustard powder, salt, and pepper as seasoning. Allow it to simmer till it thickens after about 5 minutes.

3. Put off the heat and stir till there is complete melting. Stir in cauliflower and keep stirring until fully consumed in cheese sauce.
4. Use salt and pepper as seasonings, then garnish with chives. Serve.

BEST-EVER CAULIFLOWER STUFFING

Makes 6 servings
Setting: low | Prep time: 15 minutes | Cook time: 40 minutes

PER SERVING
Carbs: 3g | Protein: 6g | Fibre: 1g | Fat: 6g |
Kcal: 320

INGREDIENTS

- 240g butter
- 1 onion (chopped)
- 2 big carrots, sliced
- 2 celery stalks, thinly sliced or chopped
- a tiny head cauliflower (chopped).
- 125g bella mushrooms (chopped)
- kosher salt
- black pepper (freshly ground).
- 1g parsley (chopped)
- 2 tablespoon rosemary (chopped)
- 1 tablespoon sage (or 1 teaspoon ground sage)

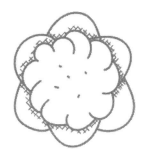

INSTRUCTIONS

1. Melt butter at medium heat in a big skillet. Add carrot, onion, and celery and sauté till soft (for about 7- 8 minutes).
2. Add mushrooms and cauliflower, use salt and pepper as seasonings. Cook till tender (about 8-10 min more).
3. Add rosemary, parsley, and sage, then stir till combined. Pour on broth, then cook till it is soft, and liquid is taken up for 10 minutes.

KETO BURGER FAT BOMBS

Makes 20 servings
Setting: low | Prep time: 15 minutes | Cook time: 30 minutes

PER SERVING
Carbs: 3g | Protein: 5g | Fibre: 0g | Fat: 7g |
Kcal: 80

INGREDIENTS

- cooking spray
- 450g ground beef
- ¼ tablespoon garlic powder
- kosher salt
- black pepper (freshly ground)
- 120g cold butter, cut into 20 pieces
- 60g cheddar, cut into 20 pieces
- lettuce leaves, for serving
- thinly sliced tomatoes for serving
- mustard, for serving

INSTRUCTIONS

1. Heat the oven to 190° Celsius and lubricate a mini muffin tin with cooking spray. In a medium-sized bowl, use garlic powder, salt, and pepper to season beef.

2. Press a teaspoon of beef evenly into the bottom of every muffin tin cup, totally covering the bottom. Put a piece of butter on top, then press a teaspoon of beef over the butter to cover completely.

3. Put a piece of cheddar over the meat in every cup, then press the leftover beef over cheese to totally cover.

4. Bake until meat is cooked through, which is about 15 minutes. Let it cool slightly.

5. Carefully use a metal offset spatula to release each burger from the tin. Serve with lettuce leaves, tomatoes, and mustard.

PERFECT MASHED CAULIFLOWER

Makes 8 servings
Setting: low | Prep time: 15 minutes | Cook time: 15 minutes

PER SERVING
Carbs: 9g | Protein: 4g | Fibre: 3g | Fat: 8g |
Kcal: 110

INGREDIENTS

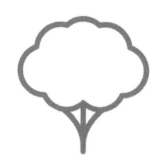

- 2 medium heads cauliflower, florets removed
- 165g cream cheese, softened
- ½ cup of milk
- kosher salt
- freshly ground black pepper
- freshly chopped chives for garnish
- butter, for serving

INSTRUCTIONS

1. Boil water in a large pot.
2. Add cauliflower florets and cook until they are tender (usually ten minutes). Drain well, using a clean dish towel or paper towel to remove as much water as possible.
3. Return to pot and mash cauliflower with a potato masher until smooth, and no large chunks remain.
4. Stir in cream cheese and milk and season with salt and pepper and mash until completely combined and creamy. (Add a couple more tablespoons of milk until you reach desired consistency.)
5. Garnish with chives, season with more pepper, and top with a pat of butter.

LOADED CAULIFLOWER SALAD

Makes 6 servings
Setting: low | Prep time: 10 minutes | Cook time: 30 minutes

PER SERVING
Carbs: 13g | Protein: 19g | Fibre: 4g | Fat: 35g |
Kcal: 440

INGREDIENTS

- 1 large head cauliflower, cut into florets
- 6 slices of bacon
- 120g sour cream
- 60g mayonnaise
- 15ml lemon juice
- ¼ tablespoon of garlic powder
- kosher salt
- freshly ground black pepper
- 120g shredded cheddar
- 15g finely chopped chives

INSTRUCTIONS

1. Bring about ¼" water to boil in a large bowl. Add cauliflower, cover the pan, and then steam until tender (should take about 4 minutes). Drain and let cool while you prep other ingredients.
2. In a large skillet over medium heat, cook bacon until crispy, about 3 minutes per side. Move to a paper towel-lined plate to drain, then chop.
3. In a large bowl, whisk together sour cream, mayonnaise, lemon juice, and garlic powder. Add cauliflower and toss gently. Season with salt and pepper, then fold in bacon, cheddar, and chives. Serve warm or at room temperature.

BACON ASPARAGUS BITES

Makes 6 servings
Setting: low | Prep time: 10 minutes | Cook time: 30 minutes

PER SERVING
Carbs: 3g | Protein: 5g | Fibre: 1g | Fat: 11g |
Kcal: 130

INGREDIENTS

- 6 slices bacon, cut into thirds
- 140g cream cheese, softened
- 1 garlic clove, sliced
- black pepper (freshly ground)
- kosher salt
- 9 asparagus spears, blanched

INSTRUCTIONS

1. Get the oven to 200° Celsius and line 1 medium baking sheet using parchment paper.
2. Cook bacon till most of the fat is cooked out; make use of a large skillet with heat at the medium level. Remove the bacon from the pan and then drain on a paper towel-lined plate.
3. Combine cream cheese with garlic and use salt and pepper for seasoning. Stir until they are combined.
4. Assemble bites: spread something around 1/2 tablespoon cream cheese onto each strip of bacon. Place asparagus in the centre, then roll bacon until bacon ends meet. Once all bites are made, place on the prepared baking sheet and bake for 5 minutes until bacon is crisp and cream cheese is warmed through. Serve.

BACON ZUCCHINI FRIES

Makes 8 servings
Setting: low | Prep time: 10 minutes | Cook time: 50 minutes

PER SERVING
Carbs: 3g | Protein: 6g | Fibre: 1g | Fat: 6g |
Kcal: 90

INGREDIENTS

- cooking spray
- 4 zucchinis, cut into wedges
- 16 strips bacon
- ranch, for serving

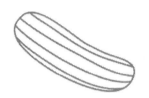

INSTRUCTIONS

1. Heat the oven to 230° Celsius.
2. Use a cooking spray with a baking sheet.
3. Wrap each zucchini wedge in bacon, then place on a sheet.
4. Bake till bacon is crispy and well cooked (it takes about 35 minutes).
5. Serve with ranch.

KETO GARLIC BREAD

Makes 4 servings
Setting: low | Prep time: 5 minutes | Cook time: 30 minutes

PER SERVING
Carbs: 7g | Protein: 13g | Fibre: 2g | Fat: 20g |
Kcal: 250

INGREDIENTS

- 100g shredded mozzarella
- 50g finely ground almond flour
- 30g cream cheese
- ½ teaspoon garlic powder
- 1 teaspoon baking powder
- kosher salt
- 1 large egg
- 14g butter, melted
- 1 clove garlic, sliced
- 3g freshly chopped parsley
- 6g freshly grated parmesan
- marinara, warmed, for serving

INSTRUCTIONS

1. Heat the oven to 200° Celsius and then line a large baking sheet with parchment paper. In a medium, microwave-safe bowl, add mozzarella, almond flour, cream cheese, garlic powder, baking powder, and a large pinch of salt. Microwave on high until cheeses are melted, about 1 minute. Stir in egg.

2. Shape dough into a ½"-thick oval on a baking sheet.

3. Mix melted butter with parsley, garlic, and parmesan in a small bowl—brush mixture over top of the bread.
4. Bake until golden, Slice and serve with a marinara sauce.

GARLIC CHEDDAR KETO CLOUD BREAD

Makes 16 servings
Setting: low | Prep time: 15 minutes | Cook time: 40 minutes

PER SERVING
Carbs: 1g | Protein: 3g | Fibre: 0g | Fat: 3.5g |
Kcal: 50

INGREDIENTS

- cooking spray
- 6 egg whites
- ¾ teaspoon cream of tartar
- egg yolks
- 220g cream cheese, softened
- ½ teaspoon garlic powder
- 1 teaspoon kosher salt
- 40g shredded cheddar
- 1 jalapeño, thinly sliced

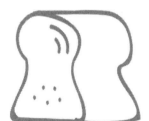

INSTRUCTIONS

1. Heat up the oven to 150° Celsius. Line a big baking sheet (use parchment paper) and lubricate with cooking spray. In a big bowl, making use of a hand mixer (or a stand mixer using the whisk attachment), beat egg whites with cream of tartar until stiff peaks form.

2. Make use of a hand mixer and a large bowl to beat cream cheese, egg yolks, garlic powder, and salt until evenly incorporated. Gently fold in egg whites and cheddar.

3. Scoop ¼ cup portions onto prepared sheet, then top each with jalapeño slices. Bake until golden and puffed, about 25 minutes.

Keto Drinks

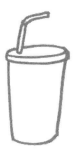

STRAWBERRY BASIL ITALIAN LEMONADE

Makes 16 servings
Setting: low | Prep time: 15 minutes | Cook time: 40 minutes

PER SERVING
Carbs: 2.9g | Protein: 0.3g | Fibre: 0g | Fat: 0.3g |
Kcal: 12

INGREDIENTS

- 24 organic strawberries, crushed
- juice from 2 lemons
- 16 drops of alcohol-free stevia, optional
- 2 litres (quarts) mineral water
- 48 basil leaves, washed, stem removed and divided
- 2 cups ice cubes

INSTRUCTIONS

1. Crush the strawberries in a large bowl.
2. Include lemon juice, then stir and keep aside. Where you decide to make it sweet, add the stevia at this point.
3. Place 24 basil leaves into the mineral water and soak for 6-8 hours. If you are skipping this step, that is fine. You will need half the basil leaves.
4. When ready to assemble, add 2 spoonsful of strawberry puree to the bottom of 8 glasses.
5. Add 2 fresh basil leaves (not the ones that were used to soak) and some ice cubes.
6. Pour mineral water over the top, then serve.

HEALTHY CHOCOLATE PEANUT BUTTER LOW CARB SMOOTHIE

Makes 16 servings
Setting: low | Prep time: 5 minutes | Cook time: 5 minutes

PER SERVING
Carbs: 10g | Protein: 9g | Fibre: 4g | Fat: 41g |
Kcal: 435

INGREDIENTS

- 1/4 cup peanut butter (creamy)
- 3 teaspoons of cocoa powder
- 1 cup heavy cream (or coconut cream for dairy-free or vegan)
- 1 ½ cup unsweetened almond milk (regular or vanilla)
- 6 tablespoons best powdery erythritol (to taste)
- 1/8 teaspoon sea salt (optional)

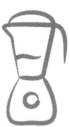

INSTRUCTIONS

1. Put all the ingredients in a blender.
2. Puree until smooth. Adjust sweetener to taste if desired.

SKINNY RASPBERRY LIME RICKEY RECIPE

Makes 4 servings
Setting: low | Prep time: 5 minutes | Cook time: 5 minutes

PER SERVING
Carbs: 4g | Protein: 0g | Fibre: 4g | Fat: 0g |
Kcal: 16

INGREDIENTS

- 450ml club soda
- ½ cup of sugar-free raspberry syrup
- 4 limes
- 170ml of gin
- 8 fresh mint leaves
- ice

INSTRUCTIONS

1. Put together limes and mint leaves in four tall glasses.
2. Add ice and club soda and sugar-free raspberry syrup.
3. Add in your liquor of choice.
4. Mix to combine.
5. Garnish with raspberries, limes, and more mint leaves.

BLACK BEAUTY LOW CARB VODKA DRINK

Makes 1 serving
Setting: low | Prep time: 5 minutes | Cook time: 5 minutes

PER SERVING
Carbs: 5g | Protein: 1g | Fibre: 2g | Fat: 0g |
Kcal: 180

INGREDIENTS

- 56ml vodka
- 5 fresh blackberries
- 20g of fresh lemon juice
- 2 teaspoons powdery erythritol
- ¼ teaspoon ground black pepper
- 5 fresh mint leaves
- soda water

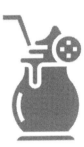

INSTRUCTIONS

1. Fill a large rocks glass with ice.
2. Combine the vodka, lemon juice, black pepper, blackberry, erythritol and mint leaves in a cocktail shaker. Crush until the fruit and mint are crushed and have released their juices.
3. Strain all the cocktail shaker contains over the top of the ice.
4. Top with garnish and soda water, with blackberries and a fresh mint leaf.

UNICORN FRAPPUCCINO

Makes 4 serving
Setting: low | Prep time: 5 minutes | Cook time: 5 minutes

PER SERVING
Carbs: 8.1g | Protein: 2.2g | Fibre: 1.3g | Fat: 22.2g |
Kcal: 236

INGREDIENTS

- 1/2 cup
- stevia
- Red and blue frozen blueberries
- 1 cup frozen strawberries
- 1 cup heavy whipping cream
- 3/4 cup unsweetened almond milk
- 1 teaspoon vanilla extract
- 2 squirts of liquid dye (optional)

INSTRUCTIONS

1. In the small blender, put frozen blueberries, heavy whipping cream, ¼ unsweetened almond milk (cold), 2 drops of blue dye, 1 squirt of liquid stevia, and a 1/2 teaspoon of vanilla extract.

2. In the large blend cup, put 1 cup of frozen strawberries, 3/4 cup heavy whipping cream, 1/2 cup of unsweetened almond milk, 1/2 teaspoon vanilla extract, 1 squirt of liquid stevia, and 3 drops of red dye.

BULLETPROOF HOT CHOCOLATE

Makes 4 serving
Setting: low | Prep time: 5 minutes | Cook time: 5 minutes

PER SERVING
Carbs: 8.2g | Protein: 2.6g | Fibre: 4.1g | Fat: 30.4g |
Kcal: 282

INGREDIENTS

- 1/2 cup hot water (not scolding hot)
- 1/2 cup unsweetened almond milk
- 2 tablespoons coconut oil or MCT oil
- 2 tablespoons cocoa powder (unsweetened)
- 1/4 teaspoon vanilla
- 1-2 teaspoons of erythritol
- heavy whipping cream (optional)

INSTRUCTIONS

1. Put all the ingredients in a blender. After which, blend until all is smooth.
2. Top with heavy whipping cream if desired.

KETO RASPBERRY AVOCADO SMOOTHIE

Makes 2 servings
Setting: low | Prep time: 2 minutes | Cook time: 2 minutes

PER SERVING
Carbs: 12.8g | Protein: 2.5g | Fibre: 8.8g | Fat: 20g |
Kcal: 227

INGREDIENTS

- 1 ripe avocado (peeled, and pit removed)
- 1 ½ cup of water
- 3 tablespoons lemon juice
- 2 teaspoons low carb sugar substitute
- 60g frozen unsweetened raspberries

INSTRUCTIONS

1. Add all ingredients to the blender.
2. Blend until smooth.
3. Pour into two tall glasses and enjoy.

KETO STARBUCKS ORIGINAL PINK DRINK

Makes 1 serving
Setting: low | Prep time: 5 minutes | Cook time: 5 minutes

PER SERVING
Carbs: 4g | Protein: 1g | Fibre: 0g | Fat: 12g |
Kcal: 122

INGREDIENTS

- 1 cup of boiling water
- 1 lipton berry hibiscus tea bag
- 1 celestial seasoning raspberry zinger tea bag
- 2 tablespoons joy-filled eats sweetener
- 1 cup of cold water and ice cubes (1 ½ cups together)
- ¼ cup full-fat coconut milk
- 3 fresh strawberries
- pinch of xanthan gum helps avoid separation

INSTRUCTIONS

1. Pour boiling water on the tea bags, then steep for 5 minutes in a large measuring cup.
2. Add the sweetener and stir to dissolve.
3. Add 1 ½ cups ice water. Stir to melt the ice.
4. Blend this with coconut milk and strawberries.
5. Add and blend in the xanthan gum.
6. Pour over additional ice and strawberry chunks.

KETO STARBUCKS ORIGINAL PINK DRINK SMOOTHIE

Makes 1 serving
Setting: low | Prep time: 5 minutes | Cook time: 5 minutes

PER SERVING
Carbs: 4g | Protein: 1g | Fibre: 0g | Fat: 12g |
Kcal: 122

INGREDIENTS

- 120g boiling water
- 1 lipton berry hibiscus tea bag
- 1 celestial seasoning raspberry zinger tea bag
- 2 tablespoons joy filled eats Sweetener
- 90g ice
- ¼ cup of full-fat coconut milk
- 4 strawberries (fresh)
- pinch of xanthan gum assists in avoiding separation

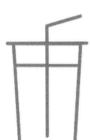

INSTRUCTIONS

1. Use a glass measuring cup to pour boiling water over the tea bags and steep for 5 minutes.
2. Put the sweetener and stir to dissolve.
3. Add ice to make this equal to one cup. Stir to make the ice melt.
4. Blend this with coconut milk and strawberries.
5. Add and blend in the xanthan gum. Pour over additional ice and strawberry chunks.

KETO STARBUCKS ORIGINAL PINK DRINK (TRIM HEALTHY MAMA FUEL PULL VERSION)

Makes 1 serving
Setting: low | Prep time: 5 minutes | Cook time: 5 minutes

PER SERVING
Carbs: 4g | Protein: 1g | Fibre: 0g | Fat: 12g |
Kcal: 122

INGREDIENTS

- 1 cup of boiling water
- 1 lipton berry hibiscus tea bag
- 1 celestial seasoning raspberry zinger tea bag
- 2 tablespoons joy-filled eats sweetener
- 100g ice
- 1 cup of cold water
- 1 ½ tablespoons full-fat coconut milk
- 2 fresh strawberries
- pinch of xanthan gum helps avoid separation

INSTRUCTIONS

1. Use a glass measuring cup to pour boiling water over the tea bags and steep for 5 minutes.
2. Add the sweetener and stir to dissolve.
3. Add ice and cold water. Stir to allow ice to melt.
4. Blend the ingredients with coconut milk and strawberries.
5. Add and blend the xanthan gum. Pour over additional ice.

Conclusion

The keto diet has become popular because of its effectiveness in weight loss and in the treatment of other illnesses. The trick to fully maximizing the benefits of this diet is consistency.

The recipes given in this book bring you a step closer to achieving your goal by offering a wide array of options to explore and choose from. However, if you ever find yourself wanting to drop out of your diet plan, just remember; the goal is worth the wait.

Disclaimer

This book contains opinions and ideas of the author and is meant to teach the reader informative and helpful knowledge while due care should be taken by the user in the application of the information provided. The instructions and strategies are possibly not right for every reader and there is no guarantee that they work for everyone. Using this book and implementing the information/recipes therein contained is explicitly your own responsibility and risk. This work with all its contents, does not guarantee correctness, completion, quality or correctness of the provided information. Misinformation or misprints cannot be completely eliminated.

Printed in Great Britain
by Amazon

76139967R00066